Mixing

Joseph McCray

Linda Ullah,

Thanks for your commitment.

God Bless

Joseph McCray

Copyright © 2013 Joseph McCray

All rights reserved.

978-0-9910386-0-2

DEDICATION

I dedicate this book to my son Goshen who has yet to experience the power of mixing, but will be ready when he does. I love you so much.

To my sister Lucille Pinkney who has heard me talk about this book day in and day out. You are such a blessing to me.

To Pastor Kenneth Robinson and Lady Lenyar Robinson, my pastors and spiritual leaders. Thanks so much for your guidance and being people of integrity.

To my wife and friend Shawanda for being the most I could ever ask for.

CONTENTS

	Acknowledgments	i
1	I'm Going to Write Another Book	5
2	Mixing	13
3	So When Are You Going to Talk about HIV?	23
4	Truths about HIV	33
5	Mixing Sexually	41
6	My Bold Friend	49
7	Goshen	55
8	Magic	61
9	Species	67
10	What are We Doing?	73
	References	77

ACKNOWLEDGMENTS

I want to thank Stephanie Rosalyn Mitchell, Mary Coupe Bekker, Richard Bush, Alexander McCray and Mia Terkowitz for your lengthy and detailed edits to the book. You definitely helped to shape my ideas into a better book. Your work was so valuable to me.

Thanks Minister Sylvester Bracey, your encouragement and inspiration early on in this project truly helped me to keep on writing, thank you. Kirk Messick I appreciate all the photos you did not like to help me choose the right one. Louty Bamba your contributions on chapter 5 have been included, thanks for taking the time out. Jennifer Gibson, classmate and sincere person, thanks for looking forward to the book. You will be blessed. Laverne Perlie thanks for encouraging me to write more on my, "Bold Friend." Liz Ellis thanks for pushing me to simplify, "Truths about HIV," It does make for a better read. Pastor Adrian Tiggle, thanks for your sincere input on chapter one, I did incorporate some of your suggestions. Dionne Waldron thanks for the encouraging words, you helped to inspire me. Thanks Stanley Pyles, Pharm. D. for you feedback on Chapter 8, you are the best. Alisha McCray, Terea McCray and Nakisha Pinkney my nieces, I want to thank you for taking a look at my photos and giving me your opinions. You ladies are so honest. Thanks Adrian Motley for letting me know that there is a writer in me. Thanks Author, Chris Kosmides for the complements on the title. Thanks to the Hampden Writers Club you all are the best editors a young writer could ask for. Thanks Wilma Brockington for sharing your trade secrets of writing. You are a jewel and thanks to the Black Writers Guild for the information and encouragement to keep, "Pushing On." Thanks Dennis Mar for your feedback. Thanks to my oldest sister Anita Camper who gave me by first collection of books when I was a kid. I never knew I would be a writer one day. Thanks Dr. Alan Baer, the best doctor in the land and for taking time out to look over my work and for your encouragement. Thanks Beatrice Grant for giving me my first opportunity to teach in 1990 and for liking the title, "Mixing." Thanks to Elders and Author Karen and Eley Gatling for continuing to encourage me. Thanks Elders Dan Murrill and David Isaac for being my big brothers in the faith. I'm running out of room, but I want to thank Josephine Jordan and Paul Neal my parents who have left this earth, but never my heart. Lastly, I want to thank everyone who has wished me well, prayed for me and encouraged me to be my best. God really bless them good.

Most of all, thank you Jesus Christ for being the author and finisher of my faith.

Disclaimer

This book is directed towards men and women of all ages who are sexually active or thinking about becoming sexually active. This book is designed to provide information about [the subject matter covered] sex and HIV. It is sold with the understanding that the publisher and author is not engaged in rendering legal or medical services. If legal, medical or other expert assistance is required, the services of a competent professional should be sought.

Every effort has been made to make this book as complete and as accurate as possible. However, there may be mistakes both typographical and in content. Therefore, this [text] book should be used only as a general guide and not as the ultimate source on the topic of sex or HIV.

The purpose of this book [it] is to educate [and entertain]. The author and publisher shall have neither liability nor responsibility to any person or entity with respect to any loss or damage caused or alleged to be caused directly or indirectly by the information contained in this book.

If you are offended by my recurring Christian references throughout this book, I do not apologize. But I hope you will find valuable information whatever may be your spiritual orientation: Christian, Jewish, Muslim, Hindu, agnostic, atheist or other. Remember, I am not preaching to you from the pulpit but advising you from the clinic. If you do not wish to be bound by the above, you may return this book for a full refund.

Chapter 1

»»»

I'm Going to Write Another Book

Joseph McCray

It is April 12, 2013, and I'm going to write another book. My first book, *Pushing On – Wonderful Stories about the Life of Josephine Jordan*, was collaboration with siblings and a grandson, introducing the wisdom and determination our mom and grandma gave us and sharing it with the world." This time, I'm writing alone. The book is called *Mixing*; it's about sexuality, condoms, no condoms, HIV and AIDS, and a little bit of my own experiences. I'll write until I don't have any more to write about, "Mixing" that's the name of my next book.

It is April 22, 2013, and I have a story for the book "*Mixing*." I meet a young man in his late twenties who tells me that he has been sexually intimate with a young lady for the past four years. He goes on to say that she was HIV positive throughout the relationship but never told him until she became pregnant. He says, "she was afraid I would get mad and hurt her." Recently he got tested and received the disappointing news in January that he has the Human Immunodeficiency Virus (HIV). The baby is almost due, and he tells me that he is so "depressed" about having HIV. His story is like many others so worthy to be recorded in my new book *Mixing – Sex and HIV*. You'll notice I have changed the title; that's good perception.

It is April 26, 2013, and I keep making these mental notes. I have the day off and I'm watching one of my favorite shows, *The Judge Mathis Show*. The story is about a young lady who is suing her ex-boyfriend because he is trying to deny that he is the father of her child. She is suing him because he showed her a paternity test that he obtained from a tax preparation company. This paternity test says he is not the father. She doesn't think it is a legitimate test because of where he obtained it. The paternity test is repeated on *The Judge Mathis Show,* and the results are the same as the first test from the tax preparation company. He is not the father of her unborn child. What's so interesting is that she was five months pregnant and sexually slept with her ex-boyfriend, then told her then-current boyfriend that she had an affair or sexual act of mixing with this other fellow. This is what prompted him to obtain the paternity test. While I watched this show, I became even more convinced that it was the right time to write *Mixing – Sex and HIV*.

Folks are having unprotected sex. Fluids are being exchanged. A life was about to come forth into this world, and the mother had no idea whom she had mixed with to bring forth that life.

It is May 27, 2013, the day before Memorial Day, and where am I? I am about to get my hair cut by Jennifer, my hair stylist and master barber. She is talking with Melonie, her co-worker hair stylist/barber about HIV and my upcoming book. We all get into a discussion. Melonie believes Earvin "Magic" Johnson is cured of HIV. I tell them that he was in Baltimore in May 15, 2007, speaking at Set the Captives Free Church, and that he declared he was not cured of HIV.[1] *Cured* means that you have gotten rid of something, it no longer is a part of you to harm you, and you are not continuing to receive treatment for it.[2] I tell them that in the late '90s, *Jet Magazine* said that his HIV was "undetectable,"[3] but the magazine did not in my opinion do a good job explaining that his virus levels were so low that testing ranges could not detect the number, but he continued to take medications to maintain these undetectable levels. I asked them, "What if there was a cure?" Melonie believed there is a cure and they are withholding it—"they," meaning the government or the drug companies. I said it wouldn't stop transmission. People would just be getting infected, then re-infected and cured, the same way it happens with gonorrhea, which 700,000 people get every year.[4] I mentioned that 1.3 million people get chlamydia every year, too, but those are curable sexually transmitted infections.[4] We want on to talk about how some people Melonie knew with the disease looked unhealthy, but Magic Johnson always looks healthy. I told her that he had said he worked out before he was told he had HIV, and he still works out. I let them know that many times when I talk about HIV, there is someone in the crowd who has a question about Magic Johnson being cured of it or having special medications to treat his HIV. Because he is such a frequent person of interest, I will have to talk about him in the book, *Mixing – Sex and HIV*, which I will start writing in August.

Mixing – Sex and HIV is a book born out of a desire to see people have a better understanding of their bodies as they relate to sex and HIV. You may ask why that is important to me. Mixing, or the act of sexual intercourse, is very important to me. But people don't stop and think about the day after intercourse. What do you do now that the climax is over? Once the thrill is gone? It was pleasurable, but short, and now it is gone. Now you have to return to life, unless your life is filled with pursuing pleasure. Mixing can get very dangerous people, because sometimes being responsible is pushed to the side while you pursue a life of pleasure. When pleasure becomes more important than responsibility, you can find yourself spiraling into an addiction in spite of the negative things that may be happening to your life. That's another topic for another day, but I had to go there for a moment.

Mixing – Sex and HIV is about sex, penis to vagina, penis to anus, or penile to oral and oral to vaginal. It's all sex. Sexual intercourse is defined as "physical sexual contact between individuals that involves the genitalia of at least one person; anal intercourse; oral intercourse; especially: heterosexual intercourse."[5] I'll expound on it in the book. For most of the book, I will be using the term **mixing** for any exchange of body fluids, mainly semen, vaginal fluids, and blood.

Mixing was something I was told as a young boy that all boys did or had to do. It was some sort of goal, a next level, a status you wanted to have. So as kids, we wanted to mix. Quite naïve at the time, we thought it was the thing to do. At first it was just a fun activity. We played this game as kids called "7/11." This was a game where the boys chased the girls, and when we caught a girl, we gave them seven kisses and eleven humps on the butt. This was such an exciting game. Where else could you get so close to mixing as when playing "7/11"? Hormones and adrenaline were at their max as we chased the girls. The boys always wanted to catch the prettiest girls. It never failed that there were some girls who always wanted to be caught. These were the girls who had a few extra pounds and were not so cute. It was played with an even number of girls and boys, and they usually kind of liked each other in some way too, or at least they were okay with giving and receiving the seven kisses and the eleven humps. Now, we all had our clothes on. We were just kids. The kisses would be pecks on the cheeks—no way were you going to kiss on the mouth, which was nasty. While this was not mixing in that there was no exchange of body fluids, it was close enough. It's funny how early on you can get introduced to the fleshy behavior of sex or to mixing. How your curiosity is peeked to explore more. We played this game prior to becoming teenagers, before all the hormones and the acne.

I suffered with acne as a preteen and throughout my teenage years. Acne was a nightmare relived each day I looked into the mirror and had to face all those pimples and the scars from popping the ones that I thought would go away if I burst them. The sad reality was that I only made matters worse, because the bacteria or germs from the pimples go to another part of the skin and provide an opportunity for another pimple to form; at least, that's what the dermatologist use to tell me to try to discourage me from picking my face. I hope this information helps some young person to STOP PICKING YOUR FACE.

Well, the doctors did all they could to help my situation, and then I met a man who announced the miracle cure to get rid of these pimples. It was a summer day. I was sixteen and my nephew was fifteen. We were walking down Pennsylvania Avenue on the Westside of Baltimore, minding our own business, and there's this grown man watching as we are walking down the street. He keeps watching us, and he begins to move closer to the fence as we walk on the sidewalk. Just as we approach him, he calls out, "You know what you need? You need to get some pussy. That will get those bumps off your face." I did not know this man. I did not ask this man for advice. He just chose to lower my self-esteem for his own pleasure. My nephew fell out laughing—of course he would laugh, he did not have acne—but I was humiliated. It almost brought me to tears, but I would not cry. The Westside was a strange part of town that I was not familiar with, so I held myself together and kept walking down the street, but I never forgot those words. He had left a scar deeper than the pimples had scarred my face.

One day it came time for me to mix, and all I could think was, *I'll show that man and the doctors how this acne will become history.* Well, the mixing did not cause the acne to go away, and that man was an ignorant, callous fool who had nothing better to do than to insult a kid. He knew nothing about sexuality, and he definitely knew nothing about acne.

This book is also about HIV and AIDS. Sometimes it is written as HIV/AIDS. They are different, and I will take the time to explain this later in the book, but for now I want to just call the book *Mixing*. HIV is a subject I am passionate about for a number of reasons, firstly because of the WILD life I have lived—"WILD" meaning "Without the Lord's Direction." It is by God's grace and mercy alone that I'm still on this Earth to be able to write this book. It is by no goodness of my own, unfortunately. I don't get bragging rights. I was a young, confused male very much interested in pleasure and did not think of the day after intercourse. Sometimes, those decisions caused me a visit to the local STD clinic, and once the status of father-to-be, reportedly. Secondly, I have seen so many friends suffer and die from this horrible and merciless disease, a disease that they tried to be silent about having even when the signs of disease screamed to the world that they had it. Thirdly, I am writing this book for all the people I have had the opportunity and privilege to care for with HIV/AIDS throughout my twenty-eight-year career of nursing. Lastly, I am writing this book to all the thousands I have been given the opportunity to teach and empower about HIV/AIDS. This book is for them.

So I have every right to forewarn, I plan to challenge the thinking of whoever decides to read my book regarding the preciousness and sacredness of mixing. Mixing is not something that should be taken as a light affair but a major step in the life of all of us. Mixing is dear to me because of all the HIV presentations, sexual transmission prevention messages, and biblical messages I have recently learned on the topic of mixing from my Pastor, Kenneth Robinson. Ask yourself, why you would want to mix yourself with another human spirit or being. What's the attraction? Have you considered the ramifications or impacts, consequences or risks? Just thought I would get you thinking. Always remember, a book should answer a question or solve a problem. I think *Mixing* will do just that. I think your awareness of who you are will be raised.

You are going to ask the question, "Why should you be mixed with me?"

Chapter 2

>>>

Mixing

Joseph McCray

Mixing

I was born and raised in East Baltimore. When I was a kid, I used to walk to the Northeast Market with my mom. She was one of the boldest, most loving country gals from Durham, North Carolina. She was not afraid of anyone. We would go to the Northeast Market to have breakfast or lunch. The Northeast Market was a collection of eateries that had a variety of foods. The place was always bubbling with fried food, bakery items, and delis. My mom would pay close attention to how the food was prepared. The preparers of the food did not wear caps or uniforms; they occasionally would wear an apron. If they stepped out of line and began to make her food unclean by touching their hair, wiping sweat off their cheeks, or touching some other body part, she would yell, "Hey, that sandwich you are fixing, it's yours. I won't be eating it after all you've been doing with your hands." Most of the time, they would deny that they had had their hands on their hair, face, or other body parts that were not supposed to be part of cooking. They would try to intimidate her by raising their voices, too, but that didn't work. She would just say it again—"That sandwich you are fixing, it's yours. I won't be eating it after all you've been doing with your hands." Then we would leave and go to another stall. All the other customers would be in awe, saying amongst themselves, "Who was that woman?"

As time passed, I would have the not-so-good fortunate of going to the Northeast Market for my mom. I would be just like her, watching as they prepared the food. It was just in me, plus I had to report what I'd seen when I got home. It just had to happen—someone would fix the food and they would place their hands in their hair, or on a dirty surface. I knew what was happening was not right. What was I to do? The words would jump out before I could really consider what I was saying. "Hey that sandwich you are fixing, that's yours. You can eat it. I won't be after all you've been doing with your hands. I can't eat that." I was nervous, but I did it. I had to.

The cooks really thought they could intimidate me. I was a kid, I know, but I wasn't afraid of them when they would deny that they had dirtied their hands. I was not going to be moved by their loud tone or their coming to the counter. I knew what my mom had taught me and nothing was going to change me. I would have to leave and go to another stall to get food, because the cook would never apologize and offer to fix another sandwich. Cooks should keep their hands clean at all times because they can transfer germs from their hands, to the food, then to the customers. There were always customers around, so to admit wrong would mean everybody had to get sandwiches remade.

This foundation was laid by my mom a long time ago, and it remains a part of me. I demonstrate what I learned as a kid during my lectures on HIV/AIDS. To illustrate the point, I take out a ginger ale and a fruit punch, each two liters in size. I show my audience the receipt from the store where I bought the sodas, then I pop them open and mix the drinks together in large cup. They are bubbling and cold. I offer the audience members a drink. Many people happily get in line to have a cup of this delicious combination drink. I take the first sips to assure the audience that it is in no way harmful. We all agree the mixture is safe to drink, and I hand out the cups. I ask the group if they are enjoying the beverage, and they all say yes.

I then ask the group five questions.

1. Did you see the drink?
2. Did you smell the drink as you were about to drink it?
3. Did you hear the sound of the drink as it fizzed?
4. Did you taste that the soda mixture was safe to drink?
5. Did you feel the drink on your tongue and then going down your throat to quench your thirst?

The group members say yes to all my questions. They let me know that all of their senses were involved in this drink—they saw the bubbles, smelled the flavor, heard the fizzing, placed the drink to their lips, and tasted it. After a few minutes have passed, I reach into my bag and pull out a thermal bottle and ask if anyone would like a drink from this new container. The crowd hushes, with bated breath and eyes wide open. No one wants to drink from this container. I have a big smile on my face as I ask them why they don't want to drink from the thermal bottle. Some people in the room begin to say, "We don't want to drink something when we don't know where it came from." There is a fear of something in this drink that could be harmful.

What they are saying is this:

1. We did not see you pour the drink into that thermal bottle.
2. We did not get a chance to smell the drink before we are about to taste it.
3. We did not hear sound of the drink as it was poured or mixed together.
4. We don't want to taste the drink because we do not feel that it is safe.
5. We don't want to feel the drink on our tongue and then going down our throats to refresh us because it might not be safe.

I ask the group, "Why do some of us engage in mixing our lives with people when we don't know what is inside of them?"

We see the person, but we don't know what their biological makeup is or who they are when it comes to their body fluids. They allow themselves to be smelled by us, but that's no indicator of what's on the inside of their body. They could have germs inside of them such as the Human Immunodeficiency Virus. We may talk to them and get a fizz, but we don't know what's really on the inside of them. We may get to taste them with a kiss, but we still are missing the true person without testing. We will get a chance to feel them with a hug or holding their hands, but it still does not allow us the assurance of who they are internally without a test of the fluids.

I tell the audience that this demonstration is the essence, the theme, the whole kit and caboodle, the main part, the take-away from my talk. I tell them never to mix their bodies with someone when they don't know what's on the inside. Get tested before engaging in mixing. Never drink from the container of the unknown.

Reflecting for a moment, sometimes we look on the outside of a person and make a determination that what we see there must also be true on the inside. If a man or woman looks good, smells good, sounds good, tastes good, and feels good, we may be convinced that he or she must be good enough to mix with, but this is far from the truth. Remember the old adage, "Not everything that looks good is good for you." A person's biological composition cannot be determined by their outer appearance. There is simply no way to know what the makeup of a person is internally unless he or she is tested. On the physical side, there are some fatal sexually transmitted infections (STIs) such as HIV and hepatitis. We used to say sexually transmitted diseases (STDs) or venereal diseases (VDs), such as chlamydia, gonorrhea, and syphilis, are transmitted through sexual intercourse (mixing) or other intimate sexual contact[6,] but now we use STI. The terms *STI* and *STD* are sometimes used interchangeably. More recently, the term *STI* has been used rather than *STD* (especially in the medical sector), because many people are infected but may not have had the infection show symptoms or turn into disease.[7]

On the physical side, there was a time in history when people refrained from mixing themselves with great anticipation for that wonderful day of marriage. This is still the case for some couples. Some couples will devote themselves to a time of getting to know each other without mixing themselves. They will refrain from mixing because it can really make things confusing and they may lose sight of the true love that can be gained without it.Blood testing before marriage came about in the '30s and '40s after an outbreak of syphilis, but over the years, as we came into the '70s, the cost of testing people weighed against the number of people actually found to be infected was prohibitive.[8] By the way, syphilis is a sexually transmitted disease (STD) caused by a bacterium. Syphilis can cause long-term complications and/or death if not adequately treated.[52] The problem is that even if your test indicates no evidence of syphilis just before your wedding, you could get the disease days, weeks, or years after the blood test; premarital screening programs cannot do much about that.

In Baltimore, there is no blood test requirement before marriage. In Montana, the bride is required to take a blood test for rubella if she is under the age of fifty. Rubella is German measles, and if passed on to a mother, it can be fatal to her child.[8]

Another concern is the making of blood brothers. If two people want to symbolically bind themselves as blood brothers, they each cut the palm of their hand and then press them together in a handshake. Some prick the tips of their fingers and press them together for this type of ritual, or some prick their fingers and allow the blood to drip into a cup of water or wine. This is then shared between the brothers. Remember that drinking or sharing blood can cause the spread of disease.[9]

People are still doing this today, but they are using vaginal fluids and semen and mixing them. Vaginal fluids contact the head of the penis and are absorbed into the penis, and the two people become blood brother and blood sister. The penis goes into the anus, and the two who are mixing become blood brothers or blood brother and sister. It's still going on.

There's another kind of mixing, and it's spiritual mixing. You didn't think I would write this book about mixing and not refer to God's word, when God's word speaks about it. Briefly, we will see what God has to say about this mixing.

"The LORD God said, It is not good for the man to be alone. I will make a helper suitable for him" (Genesis 2:18, New International Version).

"So the LORD God caused the man to fall into a deep sleep; and while he was sleeping, he took one of the man's ribs and then closed up the place with flesh. Then the LORD God made a woman from the rib he had taken out of the man, and he brought her to the man. The man said, 'This is now bone of my bones and flesh of my flesh; she shall be called 'woman,' for she was taken out of man. That is why a man leaves his father and mother and is united to his wife, and they become one flesh" (Genesis 2:21 – 24, New International Version).

Adam recognizes that his bone is a part of this creature, and he recognizes that his flesh is a part of her too. He has not named her yet, so the name he chooses is *woman*. Then we get a prophetic message for marriages and mixing for the future. We are told that a man leaves his father and mother and is united to his wife, and they become one flesh, two become one. This is mixing. Two come together and become one—just like my audiences see in that drink demonstration. Just like ginger ale and fruit punch. Mixing is from God. It goes way back to Genesis 2. The man and woman become one flesh. They are to leave father and mother and unite, become one flesh. The only way this is possible is by mixing—sexual intercourse, folks—mixing bodily fluids, intimacy is what I am saying. You see, I did not make this up. This was God's plan all the time. Adam knew Eve because, he said, she was bone of his bone and flesh of his flesh. A part of him was in her and a part of her was in him.

One more Bible lesson while I have your attention as it relates to mixing. We see an example of mixing in the New Testament. This portion of the text warns us to be careful of whom we mix our lives with.

For those who are reading this and can receive this, this is for you. This is a conversation the Apostle Paul is having with the church of Corinth. He says to them:

"I have the right to do anything,' you say—but not everything is beneficial. 'I have the right to do anything'—but I will not be mastered by anything. You say, 'Food for the stomach and the stomach for food, and God will destroy them both.' The body, however, is not meant for sexual immorality but for the Lord, and the Lord for the body. By his power, God raised the Lord from the dead, and he will raise us also. Do you not know that your bodies are members of Christ himself? Shall I then take the members of Christ and unite them with a prostitute? Never! Do you not know that he who unites himself with a prostitute is one with her in body? For it is said, 'The two will become one flesh.' But whoever is united with the Lord is one with him in spirit.

"Flee from sexual immorality. All other sins a person commits are outside the body, but whoever sins sexually sins against their own body. Do you not know that your bodies are temples of the Holy Spirit, who is in you, whom you have received from God? You are not your own; you were bought at a price. Therefore honor God with your bodies" (I Corinthians 6:12 -20, New International Version).

Verse 15 says, "Do you not know that your bodies are members of Christ himself?" This is a spiritual mixing. Our bodies are members of Christ himself. We are joined to him. We are the body of Christ, each doing our part for the unified body. Then Paul says, "Shall I then take the members of Christ and unite them with a prostitute?" (a person who mixes their body for money). "Never!" is his reply. He could never do this, and he tells the body of Christ to never do this. He is talking to a group of believers at the church of Corinth, but it applies to Christian believers today.

Paul was one of the greatest biblical authors of the New Testament. He was warning the saints not to mix themselves with people who did not share the same beliefs or they would become as one with them and take on their nature and lose a part of who they were. They would lose the very Christian beliefs they held. He goes on to say that Christians belong to Christ and that they must honor God with their bodies.

This is true for me, too. I had an experience in my church Restoring Life International Center in July 2013 where I found my eyes roaming. I found myself looking at body parts of the women and stopped myself and asked, "What am I doing?" I reminded myself to look people in their eyes, not at their breasts or their feet or their bottom because thoughts, fleshly thoughts, will come to my mind—but when I look them in their faces, I see their eyes, which are the windows to their souls. It's hard to really conjure up sinful types of desires when I do that and they also see what I'm looking at.

Chapter 3

»»»

So When Are You Going to Talk about HIV?

Joseph McCray

1. How I first heard about HIV

It was 1981. I was in the 10th grade, and Coach Neal and I were walking near Lake Clifton High School for a track meet. He informed me that there was a new disease that was killing people.[10] I asked, "What?" He told me they didn't have a name for the disease, but they said it had been affecting white gay men mostly. That was because those were the people on TV raising awareness, but it was affecting other races and sexes in the U. S. as well. We both walked and seemed unfazed. I don't know why that didn't seem strange. How could a disease be smart or selective to determine whom it would affect, especially to choose a group of people based on race and lifestyle? We would find out that we were sadly wrong about our assumptions about this disease.

2. What is HIV?

1984 they give this new disease a name. It was called HIV—Human Immunodeficiency Virus.[11] Only humans are troubled by this virus. *Immuno* means "belonging to the immune system," the system of the body that protects us from harm and seeks out any strangers or foreign things in our body and removes them.[10] In an HIV patient, this system becomes deficient, less than, not adequate, lacking. All because of a virus—a type of germ that can be harmful to our body—but different from many germs like bacteria or fungus, viruses have a way of causing our body to reproduce more of the itself as it takes over our cells. As for HIV, it takes over the T cells or CD 4 cells, the soldiers of the immune system.[10]

I promise you I will try to break down some of those medical terms that sound so deep. First, let's start with the word *cell* or *cells*. Cells are the smallest working parts of a particular body system.[12] Before there was a you or me, we all started from a pair of cells, a sperm cell from our father and an egg cell from our mother.[13] The two cells met near the left or right opening of the fallopian tubes. They were so excited to meet, and there was a mixing of the two. The two tumbled down the spaghetti-size fallopian tubes, landing in the uterus, where they would grow for about nine months, one cell at a time.[14] We grew brain cells, heart cells, lungs cells, skin cells, and all kinds of cells.[14] These were all the first and smallest living units of each organ of the body.[12] Cells combine to make tissues, which are the walls or structures of an organ or body part, then tissues form the organs and all the parts that make up those organs, then organs go on to form systems.[15]

For another example, think of a house. Cells would be the bricks (cells = bricks), tissues would be the walls (tissues = walls), organs would be the rooms of the house, then the whole house would be the body. Hope that helps. If you are still thirsty for more information on cells or the reproductive system, I would suggest checking out the really cool videos on YouTube.com.

The HIV virus uses a particular group of cells in the immune system, called the CD 4 or T cells.[16] This is a type of white blood cell or soldier that is responsible for fighting enemies that come into our body, like HIV.[16] *T cells* stands for thymus cells, because this is the place they mature—in the thymus gland located near our throats.[17] As they mature, they become better commanders to fight enemies that come into our bodies.[17] But when the T cells meet HIV, the virus tells the T cells to make more HIV instead of fighting off the infection.[16] It is a hijacking of the T cells to reproduce more of the virus.[16] The virus takes over and the body does what it tells it. Billions of viruses are produced every day in the life of a person with HIV, and many T cells are produced and used up daily to battle this constant enemy.[18] The average adult has a thousand T cells in a drop of blood.[16] The normal range is about six hundred to fifteen hundred.[16] When a person's T cell count is below two hundred or the person is diagnosed with an opportunistic infection (OI), that person is considered to have acquired immunodeficiency syndrome, or AIDS.[16] When the soldiers are at two hundred, the immune system can be overtaken by some other germ that is normal in the environment but poses no problem because a healthy immune system can easily fight it off. A fairly common type of opportunistic infection that people with HIV acquire due to a low T cell count is pneumocystis (new-mo-sis-tis) pneumonia (new-mone-ya), which is caused by a fungus.[16] We all breathe in this germ all the time, but our T cell soldiers stop it from making us ill. But for a person with an immune system weakened by HIV, this fungus can grow and fill the lungs so that the person is unable to breathe and must go to their nearest emergency room or die.

3. Where did HIV get its name?

HIV was given this name by Dr. Robert Gallo and Dr. Luc Antoine Montagnier (mahn-tahn-yay), a French virologist. Drs. Montagnier and Gallo are credited with discovering HIV in 1984.[11] At this point, I was out of high school and had no idea all this was going on. Interesting to note, Dr. Robert Gallo is currently the director of virology in downtown Baltimore at the University of Maryland.

But back to HIV, this virus attacks the soldiers of our body in a way that leaves our defense system, or immune functions, deficient or lacking.[16] It only attacks humans, not cats or dogs or mosquitos.[19] You can thank your supreme powers at this point.

In most talks that I give, there is somebody who wants to know where HIV came from. I will answer that question, but you will have to read a little further.

I want to keep in the vein of HIV. The virus would get into the body through blood transfusions in the early '80s because we had no way to test for it. There was only a questionnaire from the Red Cross given out whenever a person would donate blood. The questions went like this:

1. Have ever used needles to take drugs, steroids, or anything not prescribed by your doctor?
2. Are you a male who has had sexual contact with another male, even once, since 1977?
3. Have you ever taken money, drugs, or other payment for sex since 1977?
4. Do you have AIDS symptoms such as:

- fever

- unexplained weight loss (ten pounds or more in less than two months)
- night sweats
- blue or purple spots in your mouth or on your skin
- white spots or unusual sores in your mouth
- lumps in your neck, armpits, or groin, lasting longer than one month
- diarrhea that won't go away
- cough that won't go away and shortness of breath

It was the hope that people would be honest and not donate blood if they fell in the high-risk group.[20]

We did not get HIV testing for blood until 1985—what a long time, folks.[11] The blood supply today is the safest ever,[21] but sometimes people mix their bodily fluids when they share needles. Needle sharing is a sure way to obtain HIV, because the virus travels through the blood. The greatest quantity of the virus is in blood.[22] I often tell audiences that if you have two people, one needle, and one drug, you have a dilemma. If the two people both want that drug the same way, they will have to share that drug with each other, thus infecting one another. An audience member would yell out at times, "I'm going first," meaning "I will inject myself before letting someone else use the needle." That's smart of them, but that's also cocky, because it means they believe that they are without infection. They could be the one infected with HIV and could be passing it on to the next person.

4. HIV is in more fluids

* Penis

Along with blood, semen has HIV in it, as does pre-ejaculate or pre-cum. It is the second-most-concentrated fluid that contains HIV.[22] A man with HIV can pass the virus from his penis into another person's rectum. The rectum is a delicate area of the body lined with mucosal or pink soft tissue, like the tissue in your gums. This part of the body can become damaged when a penis is introduced into it. I know you are saying, "But my partner uses a lot of lubricant." You still need to know that small tears to the rectum can still take place and provide an entry for the virus when you have unprotected sex, and HIV sitting in the rectum can be absorbed into the mucosal lining or the pink tissue like our gums.[22] This has been and remains the most common route of transmission of HIV since the epidemic began in America.[23]

A man with HIV can pass the virus from his penis into another person's vagina.[22] The virus is in semen and during intercourse is ejaculated into the vagina. That seems pretty simple. Semen into the vagina could mean pregnancy, and it could also mean infection with HIV; either way, the fluid is powerful enough to change your life completely. The pink tissue in the vagina can absorb HIV.[22] You don't need a tear in the vaginal walls for HIV to go from the vagina into your body. This is the most common way HIV is transmitted throughout the world.[22]

A man with HIV can pass the virus from his penis into another person mouth.[22] HIV in semen can pass into the mouth and be absorbed into the gums. The Centers for Disease Control and Prevention in Atlanta know that transmission happens this way because sometimes an infected person reports that this is the only sexual practice that they do. When you have a person who engages in several sexual practices, it can become challenging to determine how they got HIV.

* Vagina

A woman with HIV can pass the virus from her vaginal fluids into another person's penis.[22] This can happen as vaginal fluids come into contact with the penis during the sexual act. There is an enlargement of the penis during the sexual climax just before semen is ejaculated, and tiny blood vessels sometimes break during this moment, allowing the virus to enter.[24] These tears are microscopic, too small to see with the naked eye. It could be happening right before you. Another way in is through the small tube coming from the penis called the urethra (u-re-thra), sometimes referred to as the pee hole; if you were to peel the skin back, you will see that it is pink. This is very delicate tissue and it can absorb HIV from the vaginal fluids of a person you are mixing with. For men who are uncircumcised, the risk is greater, because the skin folds over the penis and traps the fluids. This allows the virus more time in an environment that is ideal for HIV to enter into the man's body through his penis.[25]

Female-to-female transmission of HIV appears to be a rare occurrence. However, there are case reports of female-to-female transmission of HIV. The well-documented risk of female-to-male transmission of HIV shows that vaginal secretions and menstrual blood may contain the virus and that mucous membrane (e.g., oral, vaginal) exposure to these secretions has the potential to lead to HIV infection.[22]

*Anus

When someone with HIV allows someone to place his penis inside of their rectum, they can infect him or her with HIV.[22] As I explained earlier, the rectum easily tears and provides the virus an entry. To remind you, it doesn't matter how much lubricant you or your partner use; the tears are tiny and you probably won't notice them at all. The tissue lining the rectum can also absorb the virus into the bloodstream.[22]

When someone with HIV allows someone to place their tongue inside of the rectum, that is called anilingus.[28] There have been no cases reported of transmission, or getting HIV, from this practice.[29]

*Mouth

When someone with HIV places their mouth on a person's penis and mixes fluids with them, this does not seem to spread HIV. There has not been a single case reported of HIV being transmitted this way.[22] It seems like it should have happened, but while HIV is present in saliva, the amount is very low—not enough to transmit the virus to another.[22]

Similarly, no cases have been reported of HIV being spread when someone with HIV places their tongue into another person's mouth.[22] What about deep kissing, back of the throat kissing? Nope, no cases reported. However, people who are kissing like this also often engage in another, higher-risk sexual act of mixing, as stated previously. So the kissing is cancelled out as a means of spreading HIV by the higher or more risky sexual acts.

Just like with mouth-to-penis contact, when someone with HIV places their mouth or tongue into another person's vagina, it doesn't seem to spread the virus. There has never been a case of transmission recorded. The same goes for when someone with HIV places their mouth or tongue into another person's anus—no recorded transmissions.

*Mother to child or vertical transmission

A woman can pass HIV to her child. It is not clear why it does not happen 100% of the time, but it happens about 25% of the time if the woman has received no treatment with HIV medications. That means if a mother had four children without HIV medications to reduce the amount of virus in her body before the children were born, one out these four children would be born with HIV. That number is much lower in the USA, because women are encouraged to be tested for the children's sake, and if a mom is infected with HIV, she is offered medications during the last trimester of the pregnancy. These HIV medications are not harmful to the unborn child and reduce the chances of the child being born with HIV to 1-2%, which means if the woman had 100 children, only one or two of them would be infected with HIV. In other words, no cases of mother-to-child transmission of HIV should take place in the USA if the mothers get into care.[30]

5. Where did it come from?

HIV is not a man-made disease. There are people out there who think that a segment of society sat down and concocted a plan to destroy another segment of society. That's pretty preposterous. How could an infectious disease be so precise as to only infect blacks or whites or gays, females, old men and women, etc.? It's an infectious disease. That's not how it works.

First, we need to understand how germs operate. They operate by a cycle called the chain of infection.[31] You first have a germ, a tiny living thing that has the capacity or capability to bring harm to a person or animal.[32] Next, it needs a body or a host, a place where it can grow.[31] After it grows, it has to travel from that body to another body, so it can continue growing or existing.[31] With HIV, the cycle looks like this: HIV is in a body, where it grows; then it exits via blood, penile fluids, or vaginal fluids; then it travels via a needle or sex; then it enters through a blood vessel or skin injection, rectum, vagina, or penis; then it begins to grow inside the new person.

But where did it come from? In 1999, the National Institute of Allergy and Infectious Disease reported that there is a virus in monkeys in West Africa called the simian immunodeficiency virus, or SIV.[33] The monkeys with the virus were being hunted and killed for their meat, and the hunters would get cuts on themselves, therefore setting up a blood-to-blood transmission, spreading the virus from the monkeys to the hunters. Here's that word again, *mixing*. When the virus entered the hunters, it changed its form and became a deadly virus in us humans.[33] SIV in monkeys causes no disease and doesn't result in death. However, when it comes into the human body, it is deadly to our immune system.[33]

This is from the Centers for Disease Control and Prevention, and they will tell you the same thing they told me, so call them at 1 (800) 232-4636 and listen for yourself.

Now, the big question is how the virus went from blood mixing to sexual mixing. Well, there's one answer for that. Some of the hunters were also sexual beings. They either mixed with women or men. People travel all over the world, and some visits involve mixing with people in those parts of the world, so we cannot be surprised at how HIV went from one group to the next.

Chapter 4

»»

Truths About HIV

Joseph McCray

1. When does HIV show up in the body?

I have had some audience members say it has taken years for HIV to show up. When an audience member makes this statement, immediately I know we are off on the wrong course. During sex, HIV gets into your body immediately after the virus passes through the lining of the vagina, rectum, or urethra. Some might call the urethra the *pee hole*, a word we used when we were kids. As we aged, we learned to call it the *u-re-thra*.

The walls of our organs are tissues. In the vagina, mouth and rectum this tissue is very vascular and sensitive. The pink tissue of those body parts is full of blood vessels; it is fragile, moist and can be easily torn. This is how HIV can enter the body.

Remember, T cells are soldiers of the immune system, our very own defense system of the body. T cells normally defend us all the time. But when you are infected with HIV it begins to destroy your T cells. Sometimes an audience member will say, "HIV is dormant in the body for years." My reply is, "There is no dormancy. HIV is not asleep and will someday show itself." If HIV is in the body, it is constantly awake, launching a vicious attack day by day, hour by hour, minute by minute.

If you are infected with HIV, it usually takes from three weeks to two months for your immune system to produce HIV antibodies. During this "window period you can test "negative" for HIV even if you are infected. If you think you were exposed to HIV, you should wait for two months before being tested. You can also test right away and then again after two or three months. **If you are infected, you can transmit HIV to others during the window period even if you test negative. In fact, during this period of early infection, you have the greatest chance of passing HIV infection to others.**

About 5% of people take longer than two months to produce antibodies. Testing at three and six months after possible exposure will detect almost all HIV infections. However, there are no guarantees as to when an individual will produce enough antibodies to be detected by an HIV test. If you have any unexplained symptoms, talk with your health care provider and consider re-testing for HIV.[53]

2. When or how often should people be tested?

Center for Disease Control encourages repeat testing at least annually (or more frequently if risk behavior dictates) for patients with recognized risk factors. This includes individuals with HIV-positive sex partners, injection drug users and their sex partners, individuals who exchange sex for money or drugs, and individuals who have had, or whose sex partners have had, more than one sex partner since their most recent HIV test.

In some people, because of their behavior, they have exposed themselves to HIV. They have been exposed or introduced to an enemy. The enemy is HIV. When HIV comes into the body the body responds by fighting against it. Soldiers are formed to fight and these soldiers are called antibodies. This is what the test is looking for, did the soldiers began the fight.

If you are infected with HIV, it usually takes from three weeks to two months for your immune system to produce HIV antibodies. During this "window period you can test "negative" for HIV even if you are infected. If you think you were exposed to HIV, you should wait for two months before being tested. You can also test right away and then again after two or three months. **If you are infected, you can transmit HIV to others during the window period even if you test negative. In fact, during this period of early infection, you have the greatest chance of passing HIV infection to others.**

About 5% of people take longer than two months to produce antibodies. Testing at three and six months after possible exposure will detect almost all HIV infections. However, there are no guarantees as to when an individual will produce enough antibodies to be detected by an HIV test. If you have any unexplained symptoms, talk with your health care provider and consider re-testing for HIV.[53]

3. How often should people get repeat testing?

The whole idea of repeat testing yearly just for the heck of it, I don't agree with. When you get tested for something, there is something to be proved or determined. If you are not mixing and haven't been mixing. If you had a recent HIV test six months from your last episode of mixing, then what are you looking for?

I was at an HIV conference at the Baltimore Convention Center in years past and I walked over to an HIV educational booth. There was a man at the booth and he stated, "You ought to get an HIV test. I asked him why. He said, "You just should." I told him, "I've been tested before my marriage, and we have made a commitment to be faithful, so what am I looking for in this HIV test?" He could not give me an answer that satisfied. Later, I ran into his supervisor and I reported my experience. She said, "I'll talk with him and inform him better about HIV testing."

Always remember, people, what is the reason you are being tested? What are you looking to prove or determine? If there has been no mixing of fluids with another person, what do you expect to find? It's saddening to me that people are just getting tested, tested and tested, for what? There is nothing to be found. The body is saying, "Why are you drawing blood or why are you doing a saliva test?" There has been no mixing since my last HIV test, and that test was done six months from my last mixing of bodily fluids. The body has nothing to respond to. There is no enemy for it to fight and make antibodies. You still say, "Well, I get tested to relieve my anxiety and worry." Well, you don't need to have anxiety and worry if you are testing yourself in the right way -- six months from your last exposure or mixing.

4. Can people have HIV and never know they have it in their body?

There is a primary infection that takes place when a person is exposed to HIV.[47] A person may experience flu like symptoms but once this has passed they do not feel any different. Unless the person receives an HIV test they will not know they have an HIV infection. They can live many years before they start to get symptoms related to the HIV infection but again will not know it is due to HIV unless they are tested.

This primary infection takes place around the same time the body is responding to HIV by making antibodies or "soldiers" to fight HIV. It happens in 70% of the people exposed to HIV.[47] This takes place two weeks up to six months after exposure in the majority of cases.

There is a small percentage of people for whom this can take longer. I put this question to the test by emailing a host of medical providers. I asked them if they recalled their patients ever mentioning having experienced primary infection symptoms such as flu-like symptoms after they were exposed to HIV. The providers who responded said that some of their patients did remember experiencing the symptoms of primary infection, particularly the ones who prided themselves on living a healthy life, and looking good. Persons who did not recall feeling any changes were the ones who did not take care of themselves or who had a history of drug use. They assumed their symptoms were withdrawals or just overall feeling bad as long term drug users. All this is to say, people usually have some warning signs that their body is under attack and that an enemy HIV is living inside of them.

5. Is there a cure for HIV?

There is no cure for HIV, and we don't know if there will ever be one. While that would be great, we may be a long way from that reality. Gonorrhea, syphilis, trichomoniasis, and chlamydia can be cured, but not HIV. No one dies from those other diseases anymore. Would it really change people being re-infected if there were a cure? An estimated 15,529 people with an AIDS diagnosis died in 2010, according to the CDC.[51] It would be great if we had a cure.

6. Is HIV a curse from God?

Some used to say that HIV is a curse from God, and many still believe it. I do not agree with them. God is a loving God who cares for his creations. I think people have been engaging in behaviors that put them at risk for all sorts of things. While no one ever asked for HIV, it came into our world. You may believe it was concocted by man, or you may agree with the Centers for Disease Control and Prevention on how HIV came to be in the human body. But no matter how it originated, we must be aware of it and how we have to deal with it. That's what I'm trying to do in writing this book. I never get to share all this information in a lecture. There is never enough time.

Chapter 5

》》》

Mixing Sexually

Joseph McCray

A lambskin condom also known as natural condom or sheep skin condom is a barrier that protects you against pregnancy.[34] It will not protect you from HIV transmission, though, because of the pores in the condom. These pores are small openings that will stop sperm from passing through, but not HIV. Although HIV can pass through a lambskin condom, it can't pass through a latex or polyurethane condom. People use lambskin condoms because they like the greater sensation, but this is usually a couple that are aware of their HIV status and just don't want to be in a family way.[34]

A condom is a barrier to prevent the transmission of body fluids from one person to another. Condoms have been around since 1000 BC—yes, condom use can be traced back several thousand years. Images from around 1000 BC show the ancient Egyptians wearing linen sheaths. It's still being debated whether they wore these condom-like sheaths for protection or for ritual.[35] I believe condoms became very popular when HIV came on the scene because this was a fatal disease. Most condoms are made of latex, but if you are allergic, there are polyurethane varieties. Studies show that when it comes to condoms, despite widespread HIV awareness campaigns and knowledge about protection, 50% of gay men do not use them, and according to the Centers for Disease Control and Prevention, in 2010, men who have sex with men accounted for 63% of HIV infections in the United States.[36] Infrequent use of condoms is like not using them at all. One must be mindful to use them with regularity.

Like many of the people who will read this book, I was once young and ambitious. I was longing to find the pleasures of life, but I had a friend who pulled me in to give me a little advice before it was too late. I thought I knew how to take care of myself, but I didn't know much at all about HIV—me and my smart self. I thought it was somebody else's problem. My friend told me that this sexually transmitted disease, HIV, was running rampant. That there was no cure and people were dying from it. He told me that it was mostly in the gay community, but it could happen to straight people as well. The people most infected, he said, were men who were anal receptive (ouch!). This group was dying the most. What did I care? I was a track star and a teenager; it didn't make much sense to me. What did I care? Until I began to see the people afflicted with HIV. My friend told me that if I wanted to know more about HIV, I should contact a well-known hospital in the city which was conducting a study to learn more about the virus. I listened to my friend and immediately enrolled. I was scared, but I wanted to learn. And I did learn, because I did not want to die.

I remember going to my study visit and the investigator asking me all these questions about sexual practices. I was blown away that people did all these things—and some were things I was definitely going to try—then they began to ask me if I then had or had ever had things like Kaposi's Sarcoma, Pneumocystis Pneumonia, or Candidiasis commonly called Thrush. I was floored. I wondered what these things were, but these were common infectious diseases that people with HIV had. They had these diseases because there was an opportunity due to their weakened immune systems.

Once an interviewer asked, "What you would do if you were infected with HIV?" I replied, "kill myself." The interviewer looked at me with a puzzled face and repeated, "You would kill yourself?" Then I stated, "I really don't know what I would do, but I would not want to live, I think."

Participants in this study were asked to participate every three months. There would be really passionate people who always greeted us with a smile and gave us a lot of snacks. A well-known doctor headed the study, and he was so compassionate. I think he saw many people with HIV at different stages and acquired a true compassion that made him so caring. I remember most his smiling face as he would enter the room.

I became so informed. So aware of what HIV was, how it was thought to be transmitted. What it does to the human body. I did not learn about a cure, because there was none. I did not learn about great medications, because there were none. I later pursued a career as a nurse in 1984, and I'm sure HIV had an influence on me, and without doubt so did my friend. I often tell him to this day that he saved my life.

In the early 1990s, I began to learn more about HIV. I was working out in the county in a residential drug treatment facility. This was where I got my start lecturing about HIV. While working there, I encountered a scenario when all the ways HIV is spread unfolded. At this residential drug treatment facility, there was an eighteen-year-old black male who had tested positive for HIV. He had contracted the virus from his mother, whom he shared needles with as they used Heroin. She was HIV positive, and through the blood infected her son—stop for a minute and say, "Awful." Next, the son had a girlfriend, and he mixed his fluids with her and infected her with HIV through mixing. She got tested and was positive too. Say, "all so sad." Now take a deep breath and blow out the air slowly before you read this part. The young girlfriend who was infected was with child and would soon have their baby…now you can shed a tear if you want, because this was "just the worst." All three routes of transmission were at work. Blood to blood from the needles; semen to vagina from the boyfriend to his girlfriend; and mother to child, which is called vertical transmission.

I Love the Movies

Let me change pace for a moment. I love the movies, but don't you just hate when there is no condom nearby to show you that the couple was responsible or considerate? I mean, you have all the beautiful music to go along with the scenes, then there is this moment that they get naked, but there is no pause for when they discuss what's inside each other before they mix fluids. Oh, I forgot, that would take the climaxing moment away for the audience and the scene.

In the porn industry, they are discussing condoms use for their actors, but condoms don't sell porn movies. People aren't interested in watching a porn movie where condoms are being used.[37]

I don't have to go far to see how sex has had a major role in the transmission of HIV. Take my city of Baltimore. It is estimated that three people are infected with HIV in Baltimore every day.[38] The sex trade in Baltimore is high because of two drugs, Crack Cocaine and Heroin; people will prostitute themselves for these in Baltimore.[39] When the *Baltimore Sun* did a feature on sex in Baltimore, they discussed a few points that are worth considering.

In spite of all the precautions you can take to protect yourself, there are people who want to have sex without a condom and will pay more for the sex.[39]

This blew me away. There were men back in the mid 2000's who wanted to buy sex in its natural form. They didn't care what they got or what they gave to others.

To add, sex workers in Baltimore are both men and women, and Crack Cocaine use drives the epidemic of infectious diseases among them.[39] The effect of Crack Cocaine is short, only five to ten minutes.[40] After that, the drug effect is gone, the person hits a low emotionally and cravings or desire to use it again soar. When you have nothing else, you have your body, but you can choose to use it in the wrong way. There is more to you than a quick thrill, a pleasure ride. You have a mind with that body that has creative abilities to give to the world. You are talented. You were not designed to pursue pleasure every day of your life. You were supposed to have it for a little while, then go on to something responsible. Pleasure was never meant to be a lifestyle; the brain is not wired that way. So when you choose that lifestyle, you put substances into you to extend the pleasure to make it last. You seek this pleasure in spite of the harmful places you might go, harmful people you might encounter or harmful decisions you might make, like leaving your children alone or not going to work. Or mixing fluids with someone who only sees you for what they can get. They don't want to know your name and your interests, they just want a pleasure need met—but your awareness is about to be raised. You are no longer going to think that low of yourself. Make a decision to say no, to ask, "Are you worthy to be mixed inside of me?" This might be hard at first, but you are going to get there and remain.

There was a great falling away in the churches early in the 1990's as countless men became ill and died, right in the black church. These were prominent men of high positions who wasted away. They were on crutches due to nerve damage related to HIV, and then they were no more.

This disease had crippled our nation. We had no name for it until 1982 and it was called AIDS (Acquired Immunodeficiency Syndrome). No test for it until 1985. No treatment for it until 1987 and no cure or vaccine for it at this time. Folks suffered miserably and shamefully. The word on the street to say was that you had cancer when you were taken ill. Never say you had HIV or AIDS. You would be judged until the day you died. If you were a man, you would be seen as a homosexual or on the down-low, unless you said you got it from a blood transfusion or shared needles on the side. Women pretty much could say they received it from their male partners and receive comfort, support, and sympathy. A child born to an HIV-positive mother was in that category, too. IV drug users were already frowned upon, and this was just one more reason to look down on them, but in some ways they could and did hold their heads up by admitting that they used drugs. There was and is a great support network in place for them; they didn't need the church to crucify or condemn them. They had Narcotic Anonymous, a strong network of people who had come to realize they were powerless over their addictions and then to accept a power greater than themselves. It was not uncommon to see addicts confessing their sins and making a decision to repent and do better.

That is the brief history of HIV, going back to the '80s. By the early '90s we had more medications, but not quite the right ones. There was no prolonging of life.

Chapter 6

»»

My Bold Friend

I call him my bold friend because I had never met anyone like him before. He was intelligent, wise, and articulate, and he was infected with HIV. It didn't matter who knew. Marquette Prioleau, a former school teacher and poet, and I met at an HIV/AIDS fundraiser in the '90s. He would become my role model of an African American male advocating about HIV. He was one of a kind.

Marquette decided to step forward and admit that he had HIV and that he had contracted the virus through homosexual sex or same-sex relationships. This was committing two taboos in the black community—first to admit openly to being HIV positive in the early '90s, and second to admit to having contracted the disease from same-sex contact. How could Marquette ever return to the community? He didn't care. He had nothing to lose. He knew the disease was taking its toll on his body, but not on his mind. So what did he do? He began to fulfill his dreams.

His book, *The Glamour is Gone,* were a collection of poems about his life. He was free to be himself, and it was okay for the world to know. He took those poems off the shelf and placed them in a book. No longer was he waiting. He was getting it done.

He didn't mind media attention. He was in the paper and on television sharing stories of his life and his HIV status, advising people to get tested and seek treatment. He was a lone soldier out there. There was no African American man or woman more visible than he was at the time in Baltimore. He spoke very well, and he never let his sickness allow anyone to disrespect him. Once he was on the telephone and apparently the other person called him by his first name. He quickly let that person know this was a business conversation and that he would prefer being called Mr. Prioleau. I learned that practice from him.

At one point during his illness, Marquette was so close to being offered the new medications. He was at the door knocking, but it was too early to open the door for the newer HIV medications. This was 1992. Protease Inhibitors for HIV were introduced in 1995.[11] This group of medications would change the face of HIV, because they significantly reduced the amount of the virus a person had in their body, thereby giving their T cells a chance to increase and causing a decline in the death rate.[41]

I remember him getting his IV infusions of amphotericin or as Nurse Laverne Perlie a good friend of ours called it "amphoterrible," an antifungal medication that would cause chills during its administration. He would ask me to stay and enjoy his company as this medication would infuse into him. He told me it was horrible on his body, as he was simultaneously taking Tylenol and Benadryl to prevent the headache and chills that were about to come. Marquette would endure with no tears or frowns. He was a soldier.

Marquette died at Johns Hopkins Hospital in 1993. He was the last of his kind in this town. While there have been others who have championed the cause, I never seen anyone establish a nonprofit, write a book of poetry, speak at schools and libraries, and give TV interviews. News articles allowed his voice to be heard. In his own way, he was telling people twenty years ago to be mindful of mixing.

Marquette died before the resurrecting medications could reach the top of the water. So talented, so gifted, and so unfair that he did not get the opportunity to live on.

"I don't want to die anonymous," he said. "I want people to know I lived and how blessed I have been."[42]

In following in his footsteps, in1995 I began to work for an agency where I was responsible for assessing people with HIV or AIDS for assisted living. This agency provided assisted living to people living with HIV or AIDS. A provider would assist them with housing, food and social support. My job was to assess every person coming into the program to determine if we could meet their needs.

I was all over the city assessing people as they left hospitals, nursing homes, their homes and at their drug treatment centers. It didn't matter where they were, I was there. I would also be responsible for reassessing them if they were hospitalized, and before they could return to the home I had to decide whether their needs could be met through our agency.

There was one case that I will never forget. It was a young African American male who was in his late twenties. He was so angry because he had AIDS. His HIV had progressed to AIDS as his T cells were below 200. He became very sick at one time and was hospitalized. I went out to see him and determined that he could not return to the provider's home as he now needed skilled nursing care at a nursing home. Well, the provider didn't take that too well, and I had to speak on a three-way call with my supervisor and the provider informing her that he could not return. This was a first, because most people returned to her home, no matter their condition. I'm not sure if she cared that much for the people or for the income she received for having them under her care, but it didn't matter, she was not going to have this young man in her home.

I documented clearly how his medical needs would not be served at her home and how he would best be served at a skilled nursing facility. As it turned out, he did get transferred to a skilled nursing facility. I went by that facility to visit him. He didn't know I was there, but as I watched him sleep so peacefully in his room, I wanted to cry, but I didn't. My heart was so inspired and I felt that he was in the best place.

This job required me to be an HIV expert, as I encountered so many different people in so many different conditions, and I had to be able to defend my assessments. I was the one saying yes and no to a person living with HIV or AIDS. I was making decisions on who stayed and who had to go. My home was filled with all the current HIV books and magazines. They were all over the place. I attended all the conferences. I was in the know. I had to be, and what was so interesting about all this is that I did not pursue a job in HIV care—the application was for a general nursing position, but the main role happened to be as an HIV advocate and teacher.

I taught everywhere throughout the agency. Sometimes I would see people years after I had given a talk and they would remind me of something I had said to them. I was being fulfilled. I often thought about Marquette as I gave many of those talks. I thought about how intelligent he was and how bold he was. I realized, then and now, that I was carrying the same message he proclaimed years before. His message was for people to be responsible for their own behaviors in life, and that's my message, too.

My message to those who are reading this chapter is you and you only have to be responsible for who you mix with and who mixes with you. You have to raise your standard for your body. Your self-worth has to increase. You might be saying, "But how do I do that?" Find yourself a positive environment where you can grow and mature into a more positive person. Because of my faith, I would recommend church, but I know that not every reader is ready to receive church or a relationship with the Lord Jesus Christ. So you have to determine what that positive environment is that can help you raise your self-esteem, raise your self-worth as a person. Then you will be able to make better decisions about who you mix yourself with. When your sense of value in who you are increases, some people and substances will not be worthy to mix into you. You will say, "No way, José"—but it comes with work, with you realizing the need to place a higher value on your person.

Marquette did not let HIV have him, but instead he told HIV what he was going to do, and that was to live to the fullest. He inspired many, and most of all me. So this chapter is for all the people who need to increase the value of themselves, and for my bold friend, Marquette.

Chapter 7

>>>>

Goshen

Joseph McCray

Now that we've been through all this history, let's come back to the main point. This book is about mixing. As I was writing it, I was thinking of my son, Goshen. He is four years old.

We talk about body parts. He has learned to identify his penis and that it is used for urinating. At times he will manipulate it to gain pleasure, as I see him grinning. Goshen, I write this book partly to teach you that your penis is a very critical and powerful organ that God has given you. You must use wisdom with regard to what you do with it. I hope that you gain wisdom from this book and that you will apply it to your life forevermore.

God has designed you to mix yourself with someone with whom you are in agreement, someone whom you love and cherish, and someone you find deserving to mix inside your body. Mixing is that powerful. It's not something you haphazardly do with anyone. You do it with someone who has been deemed fit for you, a woman that has been fitted for you to be your wife. In mixing, two become one, both spiritually and physically. In that union of cells, yours and hers, there is a possibility that you create a new life. A child can be born from the mixing of two individuals, you and your fitted wife. We shouldn't just go out on a Friday night and mix our flesh and fluids with a person because she shakes her butt well; it should be with someone that we have deemed appropriate. If more people thought like this, then unwanted pregnancies, sexually transmitted infections, broken relationships, and violence would begin to diminish. People would see the importance and power behind coming together and mixing. It's not just a moment's pleasure but an everlasting decision between two individuals that should require careful thought, consideration, and much anticipation.

While I am not a sex expert, I will share a life experience. I remember learning about sexuality in elementary school and seeing the pictures on the screen. Teachers showed us what the body parts are and what they do. I guess because we were so young it would have been pointless to go further with any discussion, but I do remember those pictures.

At home, I never had a discussion with my mom, dad, sisters, or brother about mixing. Once, I remember two of my sisters, telling me I got here because my mother and father had been in bed together. Because I was so young, I didn't understand, and I remember getting angry with them because I thought something had happened to my mom in a way that she could not control. I thought my father had done something to my mother, making her bring me into the world. I would later find out that it was the opposite.

This is what my dad told me in 2005 of how I came into the world from their mixing. He says it was a cold night and they followed the rhythm method of avoiding pregnancy. My dad would never mix with my mom. He would avoid that, but this night my mom was not letting him go, and mixing took place, and nine months later I was born. I calculated that March was the cold night and I was born in December. I learned late how I came into being, but the story was worth placing in this book.

Today, I'm not sure how children learn about sexuality. I guess they learn in a variety of ways, some for the good and some for the bad. How they learn of their sexuality has the potential to have a lasting effect on the rest of their lives. To all the moms, dads, and everyone else: educate your kids. Use this book as a reference. That's what I'm trying to do. This chapter is to my son, who is too young to read or understand this book right now, but believe me, when it's time, I will refer him to this chapter.

Goshen, there are bad people in our world. I will refer to them as *sick people,* as they are not able to control their lust toward children. These are adults or teenagers who mix, fondle, touch, or look at the nudity of children. The problem with this is that the children are naïve and don't know they are being taken advantage of by these adults or teenagers. These sick people lure them in through play, as children love to play. Adults and teenagers play games with children, tricking them to gain their trust or trying to convince the children they mean well. They want something from the child that they do not have a right to, and that is their bodies. Goshen, they don't have a right to your body, as you and all children thirteen years old and younger are not old enough to make a decision to yield your bodies to them for their lustful pleasure. Beware, Goshen, that you never let them mix with you, fondle you, touch you, or look at you nude.[43] I will do everything I can to prevent this as well. These adults and teenagers are not well. These men and women suffer from a sickness called *pedophilia*. This means that "their attractions toward children are causing them guilt, anxiety, alienation, or difficulty in pursuing other personal goals, or [else their] urges cause them to approach children for sexual gratification in real life."[43]

When they are caught doing this—mixing, fondling, touching, or looking at nude pictures of children—they are exposed, embarrassed, arrested, and labeled by the whole world. This condition is very serious.

I want to speak to those persons who suffer from pedophilia. You can be helped.[43] You can share your thoughts with your therapist, as you can't be arrested for thoughts, but actions such as those described above will land you in jail. I hope you seek help before it gets to that point. Don't deny that you have a sickness. It doesn't matter if you are a church member, a police person, a school teacher, or a basketball player, get help before you ruin someone else's life and your own. Treatment is available.

I will provide a few scriptures that can help you on your journey. This is to assure you that God is faithful, so that knowledge can help you, along with treatment.

First, know that God loves you. John 3:16 says, "God so loved the world (meaning that God loved everybody) that he gave his only son that if you would believe in his son Jesus you would have everlasting life." If you are not ready to believe in his son for everlasting life, at least accept the line, "God is love" (1 John 4:8, King James Version). As written in John 3:16 (King James Version), "God so loved the world that he gave his only begotten son that whosoever believeth in him should not perish but have everlasting life" (John 3:16, King James Version).

Second, know that God wants you to have peace. You cannot have peace with all those lustful thoughts and lies. This peace that God will give unto you is a peace that the world cannot comprehend. His word says, "I have told you these things so that in me you may have peace. In this world you will have trouble. But take heart! I have overcome the world" (John 16:33, New International Version).

Third, you were meant to live life free. "He who the Son sets free is free indeed" (John 8:32, New International Version). If Jesus sets you free from lustful thoughts of mixing, fondling, touching, or looking at nude pictures of children thirteen years and younger, then you will be free. That's where the counseling work begins. Start your road to recovery before you are exposed, shamed, imprisoned, and deemed inappropriate to be around children.

Goshen, mixing, fondling, touching, or looking upon children thirteen years and younger is against the law and should never happen. It does happen, however, and it will continue as long as there is an evil entity in our world called the devil. This being will always use people to do his will, but God also has people to do his will, like your own father, Goshen. God uses people for good, to share a better way to live, a godly way of living. That's what God wants—to see his creations enjoying this earth he made for us, not for us to be in disharmony with each other because of mixing with children.

Chapter 8

»»

Magic

Joseph McCray

Magic Earvin Johnson. What a wonder! As I grew up watching you on the court for the Los Angeles Lakers, you were a wonder. It was like magic watching you assist your players get the ball to the hoop. You never seemed to be selfish about the game—such a team player. While I was no basketball player myself, it was fun to watch you. You made the game exciting and put joy into sports.

Earvin "Magic" Johnson was a basketball star in the 1980s who played for the Los Angeles Lakers. I liked to watch him play, as he was funny, terrific, a great basketball handler. The crowd went mad over him, and he seemed so personable on TV. But something changed in the 1990s when the team had to get a new insurance policy. This was what Magic Johnson said when he came to Baltimore on May 17, 2007, as the guest speaker at Karen and Linwood Bethea's church, Set the Captives Free Ministry Outreach Center, located at 7111 Windsor Boulevard.

I remember him coming into the church auditorium with his head held high, broad-shouldered and smiling widely. He announced, "Hi, I am Earvin 'Magic' Johnson, and I'm HIV positive. I don't take new medications for my HIV. I'm not cured of HIV. I'm in treatment, and I take Sustiva and Truvada." It was a warm and sunny day. He broke the ice by immediately addressing the rumors and myths, and the crowd was stunned. I think his introduction was like that because he too has heard the rumors that he doesn't have HIV, that he is cured, and that he takes different medications than anyone else. But he answered those questions before they even were asked.

Next he went on to say how this all got started for him. He said, "The team was obtaining new life insurance, and the requirement was for all the players to be HIV tested. That's how I found out."

When asked how he had contracted the disease, he replied, "I made some really bad decisions that hurt me and my family."

When asked why his wife wasn't infected, he said, "That's been a mystery that has not truly been answered. It was thought that I was early in my infection and the virus wasn't yet at an amount in my body where I was at the point of passing it to my wife."

Someone asked him, "How did your wife respond to the news?" He said, "She was devastated, hurt, but said we would have to get through this together."

What about you physically? "Everybody looks at me and says, 'Magic, you are so built. How could that be if you have HIV?' Well, I worked out before I had HIV, and I just continued to work out after I was diagnosed with HIV in 1991."

You must be getting special treatment—you are Magic! "I don't get any special treatment. The medications are Sustiva and Truvada." These are very potent HIV medications that were available to people in Baltimore, but because they were not as popular as Magic Johnson, people didn't really know about them. But they had the opportunity to take these medications too.

It was a wonderful privilege for me to be in that church audience that day to hear and see Magic Johnson. He was humble and just spoke the truth, I believe. He was what I had imagined him to be: a humble, honest, good person who said that he had made a bad decision but was trying to improve outreach to the community hit worst by HIV/AIDS, and that happens to be the African American people, and the church is the best vehicle.

Mr. Earvin "Magic" Johnson, you have no idea of some the hate out there about you. People really think that you are without HIV, and some of that may have come from when *Jet Magazine* ran an article about you having undetectable levels of HIV in 1997.[44] Unfortunately, some of the readers did not understand the explanation of *undetectable*. Maybe they got stuck at the part when your wife Cookie told them that you were "healed."[44] She was making a confession that through Jesus, your body would be healed of HIV. This was too spiritual for some of the readers, and some to this day have a bad feeling about the way you have been treated for HIV, as if you got some special handouts. I know these feelings persist as I encounter the comments when I give lectures on HIV. They are so mad.

They are so mad that once a preacher stood up in front of a congregation and stated that you got special treatment and resources the public did not have access to. I asked him after the service if he could confirm what he had just preached about you, and he said, "That's what *they say*." I told him he had done a lot of people a disservice by stating what he could not substantiate. Maybe they think you got special medications because actually the world was being introduced to special medications in the mid-1990s, as Protease Inhibitors were the first group of HIV medications and the breakthrough treatment for HIV. The man or woman that lived in our city who had no money got these medications and improved just like you improved, but because they were not famous, who was going to remember them after the 6:00 p.m. news? They didn't have popularity like you.

This hate for you, Magic, just isn't fair. I saw you try to tell the black people the stats:

44% of the people living with HIV/AIDS in the US are people who have the same color as you and I, but we only make up 14% of the population, according to the 2010 CDC estimates. African American women are the highest group of females infected with HIV. Furthermore, African American men make up the highest number of people infected with HIV, and most of the cases are men who have sex with men.[45]

I heard you telling us to get tested and be responsible. To stop trying to blame others, but accept responsibility for ourselves. I heard you, but did they hear you? Or are we still mad at you, Mr. Magic Johnson?—who, by the way, is living a wonderful, prosperous life and still pours time and money into the African American communities to help reduce the number of infections by encouraging us as a people to get tested. It is no longer a just a white man's problem.

I do hope people get this, Mr. Magic Johnson. You admitted to making a bad decision by becoming infected with HIV. You admitted to your wife and the world, and you didn't have to. You gave interviews, they wrote stories about you. You gave your time and money to make things better. This was for all people, but especially people that look like you and me. We have to grow up. Accept responsibility for our own lives. Whom have you mixed with? Did you both get tested before you mixed your body fluids? When will you get on with your lives? When are you going to stop telling the story that Mr. Magic Johnson got special treatment? He is not special. There is no proof he got something special. He is not cured, by his own admission. He takes medications daily. He works out in the gym. He lives his life just like anyone who has a chronic disease—he sees the doctor, takes his medications, and tries to live the best life he can. That's not magic, it's just life!

Chapter 9

>>>>

Species

I'm a big movie goer, have been since I was a teenager. Back in 1998, I saw the movie *Species II*. It was a movie about an alien who posed as a male who wanted to populate the Earth with his alien species. The way he went about it was mixing with our females. He would meet females and mix his alien fluids with their human fluids, and pregnancy would always take place. He would sometimes get the opportunity to mix with the female for free, and other times he would pay for the mixing.[46]

But no matter how he came to mix with the female, she would always get pregnant. This was an unusual pregnancy. The normal pregnancy growth period in a female is about forty weeks, or nine months; however, when he impregnated these females, the nine months became minutes. These females weren't able to get their clothes on before they saw their bellies rise to the size of nine months pregnant. The alien, in his human male form, would just be smiling as this horrible transformation was taking place. When the alien in her womb reached full term, her uterus and abdomen would explode, and the alien would come forth as a female or male child and grew quickly. In a matter of minutes, the alien would be a toddler. Before the scene was over, the child could walk out with the male alien.[46] Unfortunately, the female who was used to harvest his offspring lay dead on the floor. The female was ripped apart. She was no longer needed. He got his.

What stands out to me is just how powerful mixing is. This alien meets females and has the opportunity to mix his fluids with them. There are no precautions, and the results are instantaneous. He wants more aliens, and to get them, he must pass his alien seed along to the female of the human race.

I think we would see a difference in the way we approached mixing if the results came back immediately, if before you could take your shower or get your clothes on, the child was about to be born. I'm not for the uterus and abdomen being ripped apart, but suppose you had that bump within minutes—say you became three months pregnant after mixing that evening or morning. Or, on the other hand, suppose some type of sign showed up in you that you were infected with a venereal (sexually transmitted) disease. You had drainage. You got those flulike symptoms, like what is seen in HIV after you have been exposed to the virus. These symptoms usually develop two to three months after exposure.[47]

Unfortunately, many times it is weeks and months before we can see the results of this episode of mixing that we took part in, results like a pregnancy or an infection, heartbreak or a bond. (We don't want the results immediately. We want mercy.) The result of pregnancy is, in about forty weeks, a child is born. The results of gonorrhea show within one to two weeks in males and the same for females, but there may be no symptoms at all.[48] After being exposed to HIV, it takes maybe as little as three weeks or as long as six months to get positive results from an HIV test.[49]

We enjoy the immediate pleasure, the pleasure that is just for a moment. Apostle Louis Greenup, a dynamic preacher and conference speaker from Louisiana, once said, "An orgasm is a few seconds. Sexual intercourse lasts for minutes, but true love is a lifetime." You can buy all the Viagra and sexual aids you want. You are not going to get hours of mixing and who would want that? but minutes you will increase. Apostle Louis Greenup states, "Love is a lifetime." Love is one of the greatest attributes you can have towards each other, a gift that is not selfish. Love is kind, not proud. Love doesn't seek to be seen. Love suffers long. (I Corinthians 13:4-7, New International Version). Wouldn't you like to know that someone is willing to put up with you and not call it quits, but be willing to endure you and you endure them?

Love does not behave rudely. No showing off. No trying to embarrass you. Love does not seek its own. Love is not trying to be the one that gets the attention. The flowers were purchased for you and you only, not to be seen so the person could brag. Love is not provoked. You can't make a person who loves you mad at you. They will not be provoked or stirred into anger. Love doesn't think evil; it thinks good. It thinks of how it can make your life better. (I Corinthians 13:4-7, New International Version)

An emotional heartbreak, a soul-tie separation—many times, there is not a pregnancy or sexually transmitted infection. There was a spiritual union that's now broken. Spiritual union is when two people mix themselves together for sexual intimacy. The secular world says it like this: if you mix with this person, it is as if you are mixing with all the people they have ever mixed with.

I once worked with a man who was a nursing assistant. I don't remember his name, but it was in the 1990s. He asked if it was adultery if you have sex outside of marriage but you use a condom. I told him that it was adultery because of the spiritual union, but he said it was not because there was no contact with body fluids. I think this man was sadly mistaken, and I think he wanted to justify his actions by using a condom as the barrier that separated him and justified his behavior. All the courts in the land and the common opinion of people would say, if they saw this man inserting his penis into a woman or man, that this would be seen as sexual intimacy or mixing. While he would have a condom in place, there was a uniting, and this bond would get stronger as this relationship continued. I'm sure that many extramarital affairs start out with a condom and may continue that way for the safety of the individuals, not wanting to impregnate the other party or infect or be infected by them. But feelings will increase as each of the two parties continues in the deceptive act of infidelity. They may have stood before witnesses declaring to be faithful to other people, in the case of two married people being unfaithful to their spouses, or it could be one married person committing adultery and a single person taking part in the extramarital adulterous act with the married person.

Chapter 10

»»

What are we doing?

The big question is, what are we doing about our behavior? When it comes to mixing, what are we doing to change our behavior? What are we doing to be more mindful of whom we mix with our bodies? It doesn't matter if it is HIV, gonorrhea, syphilis, or pregnancy. The big questions people have to ask themselves are: 1) Is this person worthy to be mixed in my body, 2) Is this substance worthy to mix in my body, and 3) Should you be in my body? What gives you the right to be in my body, to mix inside of my fluids? If I have low self-esteem, I may believe you complete me. I may believe your mixing with me will make me feel better about who I am.

After mixing, I am just as much a part of you as you are a part of me, even if you wear a condom. Spiritually, emotionally, and physically, we have shared an intimate moment. Spiritually, we are connected, and your spirit mixed with my spirit through an act of intimacy, be it female and male, male and male, female and female, young person and elderly person, or black and white. We had this encounter. Emotionally, we bonded. This was intimate. I got naked before you. You entered me (or I entered you) in the most intimate way. Physically, you placed your fluids inside of me, or there was mixing.

We had this encounter. Was I mindful? Was I awake? Was I aware of what I was engaging in? Were there drugs or alcohol that impaired my judgment and caused me to say yes when I should have said no? Was I aware that I was engaging in a feeling or a thrill? We received pleasure, and afterwards, you don't even know my name!

Joseph McCray

References

1. Johnson, E. A. (May 15, 2007). HIV epidemic in the Baltimore-Washington Region. Town Hall Meeting. Set The Captives Free, Baltimore.
2. Cure. [Def. A. 1. 2.]. (n.d.) merriam-webster.com. Retrieved September 23, 2013, from http://www.merriam-webster.com/medlineplus/cure
3. Wulf, S. and Cole, P. (1997, April 4). Earvin `Magic' Johnson's HIV is at undetectable levels, doctors say. *Jet.* p53
4. CDC. Sexually Transmitted Disease Surveillance, 2011. Atlanta, GA: Department of Health and Human Services; December 2012.
5. Sexual intercourse. (n.d.). *Merriam-Webster.com.* Retrieved September 23, 2013, from http://www.merriam-webster.com/dictionary/sexual intercourse
6. Sexual Transmitted Disease. (n.d.). *thefreedictionary*.com Retrieved September 23, 2013, from http://www.thefreedictionary.com/sexually+transmitted+disease
7. Marie, J. STD vs STI - What's the Difference? Retrieved September 24, 2013, from http://www.thestdproject.com/std-vs-sti-whats-the-difference/
8. Shmerling, R. H. (2012, October 23). The Truth About Premarital Blood Testing. *intelihealth*.com. Retrieved September 24, 2013, from http://www.intelihealth.com/article/the-truth-about-premarital-blood-testing?hd=Medical
9. Blood Brothers. [Def. 2.]. (n.d.) *thefreedictionary*.com Retrieved September 23, 2013, from http://www.thefreedictionary.com/Blood+Brothers

10. Institute, S. (n.d.). HIV/AIDS. *HowStuffs*.com, Retrieved September 24, 2013, from http://health.howstuffworks.com/diseases-conditions/infectious/hiv-and-aids-dictionary.htm
11. AIDS Timeline. (n.d.). Retrieved September 24, 2013, from http://www.avert.org/aids-timeline.htm
12. Brain, M. (n.d.). How Cells Work. *HowStuffs*.com, Retrieved September 24, 2013, from http://science.howstuffworks.com/life/cellular-microscopic/cell.htm
13. Sperm and Ova (Spermatozoa and Oocytes) Human Reproductive Cells. (n.d.) Retrieved October 2, 2013, from http://www.3dscience.com/Resources/Reproductive_Cells.php
14. Gelder, G. V. The Human Egg Cell and Sperm. (n.d.) Retrieved October 2, 2013, from http://www.dynamisch.nu/feno/english/e8embryo4.html
15. Cells, Tissues and Organs. (n.d.) Retrieved October 2, 2013, from http://www.beaconlearningcenter.com/documents/1966_3268.pdf
16. CD4 (T – Cell) Test. (2012, March 29). *AIDS InfoNet*.com. Retrieved October 2, 2013, from http://www.thebody.com/content/art58838.html?getPage=1
17. Bailey, R. (n.d.). Thymus. *About*.com. Retrieved October 2, 2013, from http://biology.about.com/od/anatomy/ss/thymus.htm
18. Scondras, D. (2000, May 1). Maintain Your T – Cell Count, and Get More T – Cell. *TheBody*.com. Retrieved October 2, 2013, from http://www.thebody.com/content/art2752.html
19. Frascino, R. (2006, March 21). *Can HIV Be Passed onto Animals?* Retrieved October 2, 2013, from

http://www.thebody.com/Forums/AIDS/SafeSex/Q172953.html

20. What You Must Know Before Giving Blood. (n.d.) newenglandlood.org. Retrieved October 2, 2013, from http://www.newenglandblood.org/maine/wymk.pdf
21. How Safe is the Blood Supply in the United States? (2006, October 20). *TheBody*.com. Retrieved October 2, 2013 from http://www.thebody.com/content/art17014.html
22. HIV Transmission. (2010, March 25). Retrieved from October 2, 2013, from http://www.thebody.com/content/30024/hiv-transmission.html#q2
23. HIV in the United States: At a Glance. (2013, February). Retrieved October 2, 2013, from http://www.cdc.gov/hiv/pdf/statistics_basics_factsheet.pdf
24. Westheimer, R.K. and Lehu, P.A. Sexual – Response Cycle: How Bodies Respond During Sex. (2006, November). Retrieved October 2, 2013 from http://www.dummies.com/how-to/content/sexualresponse-cycle-how-bodies-respond-during-sex.html
25. Kaiser, H. J. (2004, November 16). Circumcised Men Have Lower Rate of HIV Infection Than Uncircumcised Men, Studies Say. Retrieved October 2, 2013, from http://www.thebody.com/content/art10024.html
26. Frascino, R. (2007, June 21). Woman to woman oral transmission. Retrieved October 2, 2013 from http://www.thebody.com/Forums/AIDS/SafeSex/Q185000.html
27. HIV Surveillance in Women. (2011). Retrieved October 2, 2013, from http://www.cdc.gov/hiv/library/slideSets/index.html
28. Anilingus. (n.d.). *thefreedictionary*.com. Retrieved October 2, 2013, from http://www.thefreedictionary.com/anilingus

29. Frascino, R. (2010, March 8). Analingus and HIV Transmission. Retrieved October 2, 2013 from http://www.thebody.com/Forums/AIDS/SafeSex/Q207187.html
30. Pregnancy and HIV Disease. (2005, August). Retrieved October 2, 2013, from http://www.thebody.com/content/art5532.html#faqs
31. Contagions – Thoughts on Historic Infectious Diseases. (n.d.) Retrieved October 2, 2013, from http://contagions.wordpress.com/2010/11/06/what-is-the-chain-of-infection/
32. Germ. (n.d.). *Merriam-Webster.com*. Retrieved October 2, 2013, from http://www.merriam-webster.com/dictionary/germ
33. Sowadsky, R. (1999, August). *The Origin of the AIDS Virus*. Retrieved October 2, 2013, from http://www.thebody.com/content/art2296.html
34. The Lambskin Condoms FAQ. (n.d.). Retrieved October 4, 2013 from http://lambskincondoms.org/
35. Condom History. (n.d.). Retrieved October 4, 2013 from http://www.undercovercondoms.com/condom-history.asp
36. Masciotra, D. (2013, April 29). Why Still So Few Use Condoms. TheAtlantic.com. Retrieved October 4, 2013 from http://www.theatlantic.com/health/archive/2013/04/why-still-so-few-use-condoms/275301/
37. Romero, D. (2013, September 16). Porn's Statewide Condom Law Dies in California Legislature.laweekly.com. Retrieved October 4, 2013 from http://blogs.laweekly.com/informer/2013/09/mandatory_condom_law_dies_ab_640.php
38. Flynn, C. (2012, May 24). HIV/AIDS in Baltimore City: An Epidemiological Profile. . Retrieved October 4, 2013 from

http://phpa.dhmh.maryland.gov/OIDEOR/CHSE/Shared%20Documents/Baltimore%20City.pdf
39. JONATHAN, A. B. (2007, Nov 04). AN EPIDEMIC'S UNSEEN CAUSE. *The Sun*.com. Retrieved October 4, 2013 from http://search.proquest.com/docview/406185716?accountid=10750
40. Drug Facts:Cocaine. (2013, April). Retrieved October 4, 2013, from http://www.drugabuse.gov/publications/drugfacts/cocaine
41. How Do Protease Inhibitors Work? (1997, December). *TheBody*.com. Retrieved October 5, 2013 from http://www.thebody.com/content/art12800.html
42. Corey, M. (1992, Jul 26). SUNDAY SNAPSHOTS. *The Sun*. Retrieved from http://search.proquest.com/docview/406745126?accountid=10750
43. **What Is Pedophilia? (n.d.). Retrieved October 5, 2013 from http://www.webmd.com/mental-health/features/explaining-pedophilia**
44. Earvin 'Magic' Johnson's HIV is at undetectable levels, doctors say. (1997) Jet 91 (22), 53.
45. National Black HIV/AIDS Awareness Day. (n.d.). *CDC*.gov. Retrieved October 7, 2013 from http://www.cdc.gov/Features/BlackHIVAIDSAwareness/
46. Species II. (1998). Retrieved October 7, 2013 from http://www.imdb.com/title/tt0120841/
47. Carpenter, R.J. (2013, June 13). Early Symptomatic HIV Infection.*Medscape*.com. Retrieved October 7, 2013 from http://reference.medscape.com/article/211873-overview
48. Wong, R. (2013, July 27). Gonorrhea.*Medscape*.com. Retrieved October 7, 2013 from http://emedicine.medscape.com/article/218059-overview

49. When Should I Get Tested. (2013, July 19). *TheBody*.com. Retrieved October 7, 2013 from http://www.thebody.com/content/6113/hiv-testing.html#when
50. National HIV Testing Day – June 27, 2013. (2013, June 13). Cdc.gov. Retrieved October 7, 2013 from http://www.cdc.gov/mmwr/preview/mmwrhtml/mm6224a1.htm?s_cid=mm6224a1_w
51. HIV in the United States: At A Glance. (n.d.). Retrieved October 7, 2013 from http://www.cdc.gov/hiv/statistics/basics/ataglance.html
52. CDC. What is Syphilis? Retrieved November 2, 2013 from http://www.cdc.gov/std/syphilis/STDFact-Syphilis.htm
53. HIV Testing. (2013, July 19). *Thebody.com*. Retrieved November 22, 2013 from http://www.thebody.com/content/6113/hiv-testing.html#when

ABOUT THE AUTHOR

Joseph McCray is a passionate, Certified Addictions Registered Nurse. He is the owner of Education for the Community, LLC a business he started to provide education about HIV/AIDS, drug addictions and mental illness in his hometown of Baltimore, Maryland.

He is married to Shawanda who is his best friend and they have a wonderful son named Goshen. They enjoy a life living for God, traveling, having fun with family and friends.

It is Joseph's hope that you will never be the same after reading this book.

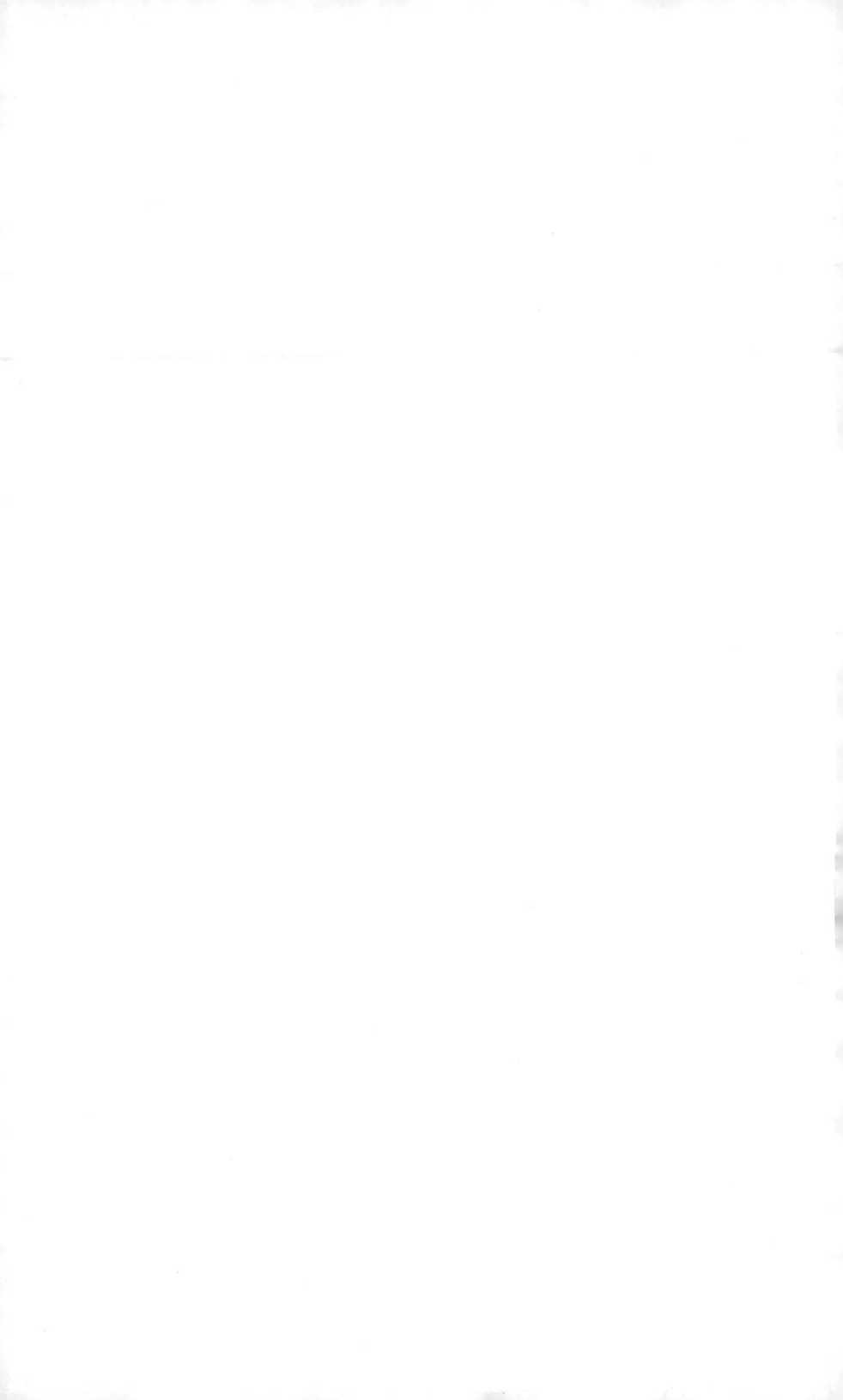